Handbook of Small
Anesthesia and An

Handbook of Small Animal Regional Anesthesia and Analgesia Techniques

Phillip Lerche BVSc PhD DipACVAA

Associate Professor – Clinical
Anesthesiology and Pain Management
Department of Veterinary Clinical Sciences
The Ohio State University
College of Veterinary Medicine
Columbus, Ohio, USA

Turi K. Aarnes DVM MS DipACVAA

Associate Professor – Clinical
Anesthesiology and Pain Management
Department of Veterinary Clinical Sciences
The Ohio State University
College of Veterinary Medicine
Columbus, Ohio, USA

Gwen Covey-Crump BVetMed CertVA DipECVAA MRCVS

Specialist in Veterinary Anaesthesia and Analgesia
Clinical Teacher
Langford Veterinary Services
University of Bristol
Bristol, UK

Fernando Martinez Taboada LV CertVA DipECVAA
MRCVS

Specialist in Veterinary Anaesthesia and Analgesia
The Veterinary Teaching Hospital
Faculty of Veterinary Science
The University of Sydney
Sydney, Australia

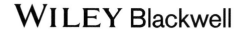

Contents

CHAPTER 1
Introduction

Phillip Lerche

Handbook of Small Animal Regional Anesthesia and Analgesia Techniques, First Edition.
By Phillip Lerche, Turi K. Aarnes, Gwen Covey-Crump and Fernando Martinez Taboada.

Reasons to provide regional anesthesia

The use of regional anesthesia as a component of perioperative pain management has gained acceptance and popularity in small animal practice over the past few decades. Reasons for this include the fact that many of the regional blocks are straightforward to perform, requiring moderate technical skill given familiarity with patient anatomy; they can be conducted relatively safely given an understanding of local anesthetic drug pharmacology, complications and side effects; and they contribute to the two major tenets of treating pain: pre-emptive and multimodal analgesia.

Providing pre-emptive analgesia by performing regional anesthesia prior to surgery leads to a drastic reduction in intraoperative nociceptive (pain) stimulation. This results in a decrease in anesthetic maintenance drug as well as intra- and postoperative analgesic requirements, thereby decreasing the incidence of drug side effects during surgery, and improving postoperative patient comfort as well as duration of pain relief. Some techniques can be continued postoperatively to assist in managing pain after particularly painful surgeries once the patient has recovered from anesthesia, e.g. instilling local anesthetic into a chest tube after thoracotomy, or injecting local anesthetic into an epidural or spinal catheter after pelvic limb or abdominal surgery.

The experience of pain, a sensory process involving the nociceptive pathway, is complex, and involves several steps. Noxious stimuli involving mechanical, chemical or thermal injury to tissue are first transduced into electrical stimuli by peripheral nociceptors (pain receptors). These electrical impulses are then transmitted to the spinal cord, where they are modulated by neurons in the dorsal horn of the gray matter of the spinal cord. Here, impulse intensity can be increased (amplified) or decreased (suppressed). Finally, the nociceptive signals are projected via lateral nerve fibers to the brain where they are perceived.

Whereas most analgesic drugs either decrease the amount of excitatory neurotransmitters, or increase the level of inhibitory neurotransmitters released in the nociceptive pathway, drugs used to provide regional anesthesia block sodium channels in neurons. This completely prevents sensory neurons from transmitting noxious stimuli from the periphery to the brain and spinal cord, or from the spinal cord to the brain in the case of epidural or spinal analgesia, thus providing effective pain relief for the duration of the block. Using regional anesthetic techniques in conjunction with other analgesic drugs that act in different ways on the nociceptive fibers (e.g. with opioids, alpha-2 agonists, ketamine) results in multimodal analgesia, contributing to an overall decrease in excitatory neurotransmission within the pain pathway both during and after surgery. This approach allows for the lowest effective dose of each drug to be used, which decreases side effects and enhances patient safety.

History of regional anesthesia/analgesia

The use of a local anesthetic drug was first demonstrated in 1884 when cocaine was used to desensitize the eye prior to surgery. Due to cocaine being habit forming and having a low safety margin, as well as the emergence of techniques allowing artificial synthesis of chemical compounds in the 1900s, non-toxic, non-addictive local anesthetics were sought, discovered, and manufactured. Initially, amino ester-type compounds were produced, until in 1943 lidocaine, an amino amide drug, was developed. Amide-type local anesthetic drugs are preferred for their longer duration of action, and several compounds in this group were discovered in the latter half of the 20th century, including mepivacaine, bupivacaine, and ropivacaine.

Principles of the major techniques

Topical application

Local anesthetic drops, e.g. proparacaine, can be directly applied to the eye for immediate relief of keratoconjunctival pain, although prolonged use delays corneal healing and is not recommended. Local anesthetic can also be directly applied to exposed tissue. Drug is directly deposited into the surgical field by dripping from a syringe, or soaking surgical sponges in local anesthetic and applying them to the tissue. Local anesthetic can also be instilled into the chest via a thoracostomy tube to desensitize the pleura following chest surgery, and into the abdominal cavity to treat pain following incision of the peritoneum. Local anesthetic cream is available as a mixture of lidocaine and prilocaine, which is used to desensitize skin for intravenous catheter placement. Lidocaine is also available as a transdermal patch.

Regional infiltration

Continuous regional analgesia is accomplished by placing fenestrated "soaker" catheters in areas that are not amenable to peripheral or regional analgesic techniques. The catheter is then attached to an infusion pump or an elastomeric bulb which delivers a set rate of local anesthetic over a specified period of time.

Intravenous regional analgesia

Analgesia can be provided to a distal limb by placing an esmarch bandage and injecting local anesthetic (lidocaine only) into a vein.

Intra-articular injection

Local anesthetics injected into joints have a long duration of action due to slow systemic uptake. There is *in vitro* evidence that local anesthetics may be detrimental to chondrocyte health, with preservative-free formulations being preferred. However, *in vivo*, this has not been shown to be definitively the case (Chu et al, 2008).

Peripheral nerve blockade

Individual or groups of sensory nerves supplying a specific region are located by palpation, electrophysiology, ultrasound or varying combinations of two or three of these techniques. Local anesthetic is then deposited adjacent to, but not into, the nerves. Nerves are typically blocked at sites proximal and distant to the site of surgery.

Epidural and spinal injection

Using specific epidural/spinal needles, local anesthetic is deposited either into the extradural space (epidural injection) or into the subarachnoid space (spinal or intrathecal injection). This provides longer lasting, more intense analgesia and muscle relaxation, while minimizing systemic side effects. Preservative-free formulations of drug are recommended for epidural or spinal injection whenever possible.

Local anesthetic drugs

Mechanism of action

Local anesthetics mainly act by blocking sodium (Na^+) channels, which prevents depolarization of the neuronal cell membrane, and thus generation of an electrical impulse does not occur in response to noxious stimuli. There is evidence to suggest that local anesthetics can also exert their activity by blocking calcium channels and inhibiting reuptake of the inhibitory neurotransmitter GABA, thus enhancing its effect.

Physicochemical properties

Local anesthetic drugs have an aromatic ring and an amine group separated by a hydrocarbon chain. The amine group can be ester or amide linked. Esters are typically shorter acting than amides as they can be hydrolyzed by plasma cholinesterases. Esters are therefore not reliant on the liver for clearance, whereas amides undergo hepatic metabolism. Speed of onset is inversely proportional to the drug's lipid solubility and pK_a, i.e. the pH at which the drug exists in equal amounts of charged and non-charged molecules. Duration of effect increases as lipid solubility increases, and decreases as the rate of systemic absorption increases. Drugs that cause vasodilation, like lidocaine, have a shorter duration of action.

Table 1.1 Clinical pharmacology of local anesthetic agents in cats and dogs

	Lidocaine	Mepivacaine	Bupivacaine	Ropivacaine
Onset (minutes)	5–10	5–10	20–30	20–30
Duration (hours)	1–3	1.5–3	3–8	3–8
Clinical dose (mg/kg)	0.5–2.0 dog 0.5–1.5 cat	Up to 3.0 dog Up to 1.5 cat	1.0–1.5 dog 1.0 cat	Up to 3.0 dog*
Toxic dose (mg/kg)	6.0 dog 3.0 cat	6.0 dog 3.0 cat	3.0 dog 2.0 cat	5.0 dog*

*Toxic dose not established in cats. Recommend not exceeding 2 mg/kg total dose.

Specific drugs

Amide-type local anesthetic drugs are preferred in current veterinary practice for their longer duration of action compared to ester-type drugs. See Table 1.1 for summary information.

Lidocaine

Lidocaine has a short onset due to its low pK_a of 7.9. Duration of action is short, lasting up to 2 h. This is due to its relatively low level of protein binding (70%), and the fact that it is a potent vasodilator. Lidocaine formulated with epinephrine has a longer duration of action due to the vasoconstriction epinephrine causes. Lidocaine is less toxic than other amide-type drugs if administered intravenously (IV), and can be administered IV to treat pain systemically, as well as to treat ventricular dysrhythmias.

Mepivacaine

Mepivacaine has a low pK_a of 7.6, and therefore a rapid onset of action. It is highly protein bound (95%), resulting in a duration of action of 6–8 h.

Bupivacaine

Bupivacaine has a pK_a of 8.1 and is highly protein bound (95%), resulting in a longer duration of action (6–8 h). The margin of safety is the lowest when compared to lidocaine, mepivacaine, and ropivacaine.

Ropivacaine

Ropivacaine has physicochemical properties similar to bupivacaine, and therefore has a similar onset and duration of action. Other local anesthetics are synthesized as racemic mixtures, whereas ropivacaine is a pure S-enantiomer, and has a wider margin of safety than bupivacaine.

Combination of drugs

Lidocaine and bupivacaine can be mixed in a 1:1 ratio to take advantage of lidocaine's shorter onset and bupivacaine's longer duration of action.

Additives to local anesthetics

Other drugs can be added to local anesthetics to enhance or extend blockade, or to decrease the pain experienced on injection.

Opioids

Opioids, particularly preservative-free morphine, are commonly administered with local anesthetics for epidural or spinal analgesia. This produces additive or synergistic multimodal analgesic effects, with analgesia lasting up to 24 h, far longer than with individual drug therapy. Complications of adding opioids include respiratory depression, particularly if high doses or volumes are used, urinary retention, vomiting (in conscious dogs), and pruritus. Myoclonus, hindlimb paresis, altered proprioception, and hyperesthesia are rare complications.

Alpha-2 adrenoceptor agonists

Agonism of pre- and postsynaptic alpha-2 receptors in the pain pathway results in analgesia. Xylazine (0.25 mg/kg) and medetomidine (15 µg/kg) have been used epidurally in dogs, with medetomidine providing analgesia for up to 8 h. Side effects included bradycardia and hypertension. Dexmedetomidine produces analgesia in a dose-dependent manner when given intrathecally and epidurally in dogs.

Ketamine

Ketamine most likely produces its analgesic effects when administered epidurally by blocking NMDA channels. Ketamine also blocks some sodium and potassium channels, thus decreasing propagation of nociceptive signals. Effective doses are 1–3 mg/kg. Side effects include increased heart rate, blood pressure, and myocardial work.

Epinephrine (adrenaline)

Epinephrine can be added to local anesthetic at a concentration of 5 µg/mL. Deposition of the combination results in local vasoconstriction, which leads to decreased systemic uptake and prolongation of blockade. This delayed uptake also results in fewer systemic side effects due to decreased plasma concentration of local anesthetic. Epinephrine should not be used when performing a Bier block or a ring block, as nerve ischemia may occur.

Sodium bicarbonate

Addition of sodium bicarbonate at 1 mEq per 10 mL of local anesthetic increases the amount of active (non-ionized) drug present, increasing diffusion across the cell membranes of neurons. This may lead to a shorter onset and longer duration of blockade. Pain experienced on injection of local anesthetic in the conscious patient is also decreased by addition of sodium bicarbonate. Sodium bicarbonate should not be added to bupivacaine or ropivacaine as precipitation will occur.

Hyaluronidase

Hyaluronidase improves permeability of tissue by depolymerizing hyaluronic acid, resulting in better spread of local anesthetic. It can be added at 3.75 IU per mL of local anesthetic to enhance the quality of blockade. Due to the enhanced permeability, duration may be decreased and toxicity increased due to increased systemic absorption. Adding hyaluronidase to ropivacaine does not enhance spread.

Equipment

Syringes

Due to the variety of sizes of dogs, a variety of sizes of syringes ranging from 1 mL to 20 mL should be available. Glass syringes, or specially made low-resistance plastic syringes, are useful when performing epidural techniques to check for loss of resistance. A specific type of syringe, called an Episure™ syringe, has been evaluated in people as an alternative to glass syringes when performing epidural anesthesia. This syringe features a compression spring, which supplies a constant pressure when attached to a needle. The operator can advance the needle using both hands, rather than one hand, allowing for steadier needle advancement and a visual sign that the epidural space has been entered (Riley & Carvalho, 2007).

Needles

Hypodermic needles ranging from 25 Ga to 20 Ga and 2–5 cm are used to perform many local nerve blocks.

Epidural/spinal needles are used when performing epidural or spinal analgesia. These needles have a sharp bevel and incorporate a stilette to avoid depositing tissue cores within the epidural or spinal space. These needles are available in a range of gauges (18, 20, and 22 Ga) and lengths (3.8, 6.3, and 9.0 cm).

A modified spinal needle, or Tuohy needle, is slightly curved at the tip, which facilitates advancement of the catheter when placing it in the epidural space. This type of needle is usually marked in increments of 1 cm along its length to assist with determining how far to insert the catheter. Tuohy needles are typically of larger gauge (16 and 18 Ga) than standard epidural needles in order to place the catheter more easily, although this may hinder placement in small patients.

Epidural catheter kits

Sterilized kits for placing epidural catheters are available commercially. They typically include a Tuohy needle, a loss of resistance syringe, a radiopaque catheter with guidewire, a connector, and an antibacterial filter. Some kits also include a sterile pen, which is used to mark on the catheter the distance it should be advanced through the Tuohy needle.

Nerve locators

Nerve locators are used to improve accuracy of local anesthetic deposition, decrease local anesthetic dose required, and limit side effects.

Peripheral nerve stimulators

Peripheral nerve stimulators (PNS) are used in conjunction with Teflon-coated needles, which have a small conductive area at the tip, to locate nerves using an electrical current (Figure 1.1). The Teflon coating ensures that only the tip of the needle transmits the electrical current so that a high current density is achieved. The reader is advised to refer to the instruction leaflet enclosed with the peripheral nerve stimulator.

Briefly, the positive lead (anode) is attached to the skin by means of a sticky electrode (ECG pad) and the negative lead (cathode) is connected to the needle. Anatomical landmarks are palpated and the needle is inserted through the skin. The needle is advanced until it is in close proximity to the nerve. The operator then turns the nerve stimulator on, setting a current of 1.0–2.0 mA, pulse frequency 1–2 Hz and

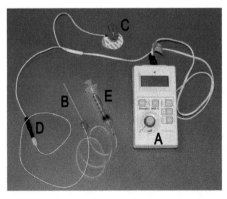

Figure 1.1 A, Peripheral nerve stimulator. B, Teflon-coated needle. C, Positive lead (anode) and sticky electrode (ECG pad). D, Negative lead (cathode). E, Syringe, injection port, and tubing. Reproduced with permission from The Ohio State University.

duration 0.1–0.3 msec. This generates an electrical field adjacent to the nerve, resulting in depolarization and muscle contraction, or twitches. The current required to elicit a twitch increases exponentially as the distance between the nerve and the needle increases. The current is reduced to the lowest possible setting required to elicit a twitch, and this is done whilst carefully redirecting the needle so that it is in close proximity to the nerve. The useful current is not a painful stimulus, and can be used in a sedated patient. Once the lowest possible current required to elicit a twitch has been determined, local anesthetic is injected through the needle via tubing. Injection of local anesthetic pushes the needle a little further away from the nerve, so twitches are usually diminished or lost immediately after injection.

Ultrasound

Ultrasound probes can be used to visualize nerves directly both prior to and during needle placement and anesthetic drug deposition, which allows for improved accuracy of blockade. This technique is often combined with a nerve stimulator to confirm nerve location, allowing drug deposition close to, but not into, the nerve.

Differential pressure transducer

The likelihood of injury to nerves during local anesthetic injection is increased when injections are performed under high pressure. The use of an in-line pressure transducer allows consistent force to be applied during injection.

Acoustic device

Identification of needle entry into, or puncture of, the epidural space can be difficult using the conventional loss of resistance technique. Acoustic amplification has been used to detect puncture more accurately. An in-line pressure transducer is attached to a pressure amplifier, which in turn is attached to a loudspeaker. The sound of the needle passing from low resistance surrounding tissues to the high resistance of the ligamentum flavum can be appreciated audibly (Lechner et al, 2002).

Complications and contraindications

In general safe practice, knowing when a local anesthetic technique is contraindicated is essential, as is an understanding of the complications of local anesthetic administration and how to treat them.

Complications can be broadly categorized as local or systemic problems.

Local

Skin
Local analgesic techniques should not be attempted where the skin overlying the site of injection is inflamed, infected, or clearly neoplastic as this may promote transmission and spread of infectious organisms or neoplastic cells into adjacent tissue.

Nerve
Direct trauma to nerves from the needle or high-pressure injection may result in loss of sensation, pain, discomfort and/or motor weakness that may be temporary, lasting days to years, or permanent. Damage to blood vessels close to nerves, particularly those with poor blood supply, may lead to ischemia. Finally, local anesthetic drugs or additives may be directly toxic to nervous tissue.

Systemic

Central nervous system
Excessive systemic uptake of local anesthetic can cause seizures. This occurs because inhibitory neurons are more sensitive to Na^+ channel blockade, and if they are blocked then excitation results.

Cardiovascular
Local anesthetic techniques should be performed with caution or avoided in patients that are hypotensive or in shock, as inadvertent drug administration into a vein or unexpected rapid systemic drug absorption may lead to cardiovascular collapse.

Coagulopathy
Techniques in which hemorrhage is a possible complication, e.g. epidural block, should not be performed in patients where coagulopathy has been demonstrated or is suspected. Laceration of a blood vessel may lead to bleeding that will be hard to control. If uncontrolled hemorrhage occurs in a closed space, it may lead to pressure necrosis of adjacent tissues.

Species differences and considerations

As a species, cats are generally less amenable to being restrained for procedures unless they are heavily sedated or anesthetized, compared to dogs in which some techniques can be performed with light sedation. It can also be more challenging to accurately weigh cats, which may lead to inadvertent under- or overdosage. Regardless of species, accurate dosing will lead to fewer complications. Inhalant anesthesia with isoflurane or sevoflurane decreases metabolism of lidocaine after 2 mg/kg intravenous administration in cats, even at relatively low inhalant doses, whereas this is not the case in dogs (Thomasy et al, 2005). Rapid inadvertent intravenous injection of lidocaine, while not ideal in any species, may be more problematic in cats.

Safe practice

Gaining confidence

Local anesthetic techniques vary in their level of difficulty to perform, effectiveness of block, and complexity of equipment required. Starting by using straightforward techniques that require little in the way of extra equipment, and have been reported to have high success rates, is recommended. Once comfortable with simple techniques, the practitioner can expand his or her repertoire. Attending continuing education seminars and courses on local anesthetic techniques, particularly when a wet lab is a component of the training, is recommended. We also believe that using this book will be an asset when it comes to performing techniques where the practitioner has little or no experience.

Making a plan

Regardless of technique, successfully performing local anesthetic blocks requires preparation of the appropriate equipment, and a thorough understanding of patient anatomy and local anesthetic drug pharmacology. It is also important that the clinician performing the local anesthetic block has an appreciation of the potential complications that might occur and is able to develop a plan to treat them (see Chapter 7). The person performing the block should also have in mind an alternative plan for providing analgesia should the block prove impossible to perform, or in cases where continuing with the block is contraindicated (e.g. severe drop in blood pressure during epidural administration, skin infection over injection site becomes apparent after clipping).

References

Chu, C.R., Izzo, N.J., Coyle, C.H., et al. (2008) The in vitro effects of bupivacaine on articular chondrocytes. *J Bone Joint Surg* **90**: 814–820.

Lechner, T.J.M., van Wijk, M.G.F. & Maas, J.J. (2002) Clinical results with a new acoustic device to identify the epidural space. *Anaesthesia* **57**: 768–772.

Riley, E.T. & Carvalho, B. (2007) The Episure syringe: a novel loss of resistance syringe for locating the epidural space. *Anesth Analg* **105**: 1164–1166.

Thomasy, S.M., Pypendop, B.H., Ilkiw, J.E. & Stanley, S.D. (2005) Pharma-cokinetics of lidocaine and its active metabolite, monoethylglycinexylidide, after intravenous administration of lidocaine to awake and isoflurane-anesthetized cats. *Am J Vet Res* **66**: 1162–1166.

Further reading

Campoy, L. & Read, M.R. (2013) *Small Animal Regional Anesthesia and Analgesia*. Ames, IA: Wiley-Blackwell.

Shelby, A.M. & McKune, C.M. (2014) *Small Animal Anesthesia Techniques*. Ames, IA: Wiley-Blackwell.

Tranquilli, W.J., Thurmon, J.C. & Grimm, K.A. (2007) *Lumb & Jones Veterinary Anesthesia*, 4th edn. Ames, IA: Wiley-Blackwell.

CHAPTER 2

Cutaneous Innervation Index

Gwen Covey-Crump

Handbook of Small Animal Regional Anesthesia and Analgesia Techniques, First Edition.
By Phillip Lerche, Turi K. Aarnes, Gwen Covey-Crump and Fernando Martinez Taboada.
© 2016 John Wiley & Sons, Ltd. Published 2016 by John Wiley & Sons, Ltd.

Cutaneous innervation index

Use this chapter as an aid to choosing an appropriate regional anesthetic technique for the planned procedure.

Canine dermatomes – Body

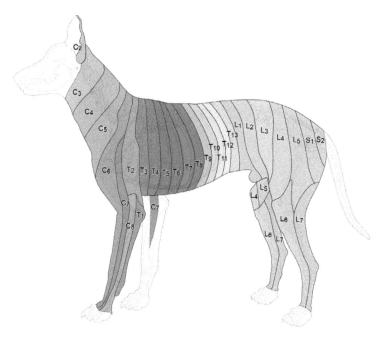

Figure 2.1 Canine dermatome map. Cutaneous innervation according to spinal segment. This is intended as a guide only as much overlap between segments and variation between animals exist. Redrawn from Oliver, J.E. & Lorenz, M.D. (eds) (1983) *Veterinary Neurologic Diagnosis*. Philadelphia: W.B.Saunders Co. Reproduced with permission from The Ohio State University.

Head

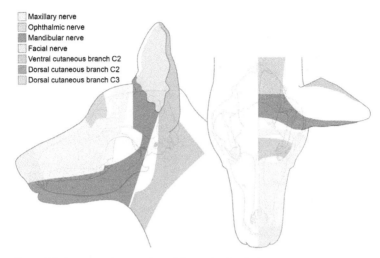

Figure 2.2 Cutaneous innervation of the canine head. Autonomous sensory regions are shown. Some overlap and variation between zones and animals exist. Reproduced with permission from The Ohio State University.

Thoracic limb

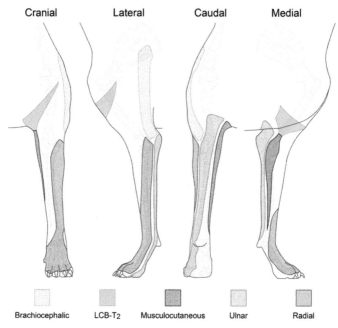

Figure 2.3 Cutaneous innervation of the canine thoracic limb. Autonomous sensory regions are shown. Some overlap and variation between zones and animals exist. LCB-T_2, lateral cutaneous brachial nerve-thoracic 2. Reproduced with permission from The Ohio State University.

Table 2.1 Sensory innervation of the canine thoracic limb

	Region	Nerve	Techniques
C6–7	Lateral shoulder and joint	Suprascapular	CP
		Subscapular	CP
C7–8	Craniomedial antebrachium	Musculocutaneous	CP, BP, RUMM
C8	Caudal shoulder joint, lateral brachium	Axillary	CP, BP
C7–T1	Lateral elbow joint, craniolateral antebrachium, carpus and digits	Radial	CP, BP, RUMM
C8–T1	Medial elbow joint	Median	CP, BP, RUMM
C8–T2	Caudal elbow joint, caudolateral antebrachium, carpus and digits	Ulnar	CP, BP, RUMM

BP, brachial plexus; CP, cervical paravertebral; RUMM, radial, ulnar, median, musculocutaneous.

Pelvic limb

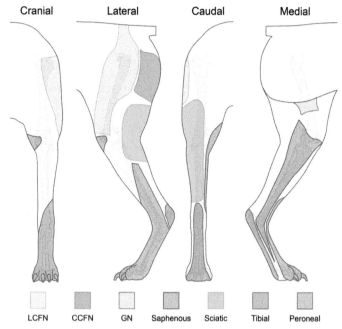

Figure 2.4 Cutaneous innervation of the canine pelvic limb. Autonomous sensory regions are shown. Some overlap and variation between zones and animals exist. Reproduced with permission from The Ohio State University.

Table 2.2 Sensory innervation of the canine pelvic limb

	Region				Techniques
L4	Hemipelvis (excl. skin overlying hip joint), medial thigh, stifle, leg, hock		Femoral	Saphenous	Inguinal
L5					Preiliac
L6					Psoas compartment
L7	Entire limb distal to stifle (excl. medial strip)	Dorsolateral distal limb	Sciatic	Peroneal	Lateral Parasacral Transgluteal
S1, S2		Laterocaudal distal limb		Tibial	

CHAPTER 3

Infiltration Blocks

Fernando Martinez Taboada

Handbook of Small Animal Regional Anesthesia and Analgesia Techniques, First Edition.
By Phillip Lerche, Turi K. Aarnes, Gwen Covey-Crump and Fernando Martinez Taboada.
© 2016 John Wiley & Sons, Ltd. Published 2016 by John Wiley & Sons, Ltd.

Infiltration for mass removal

Line and ring blocks

Indications
Surgical resection of cutaneous or superficial masses, surgical closure of lacerations, procedures involving an appendage (e.g. toe, tail, pinna, etc.)

Target nerves
Cutaneous nerves of the affected area

Region anesthetized
Appendage distal to the block, area immediately underneath the block and, in the case of performing a ring block, area circumscribed by it

Landmarks
Surrounding tissue around the area of interest. It is fundamental that the subcutaneous tissue is clearly identified

Needle
Hypodermic needle. It is recommended to use a longer length but small in size needle (e.g. 23 Ga 2.5–3.8 cm)

Depth
Subcutaneous injection of local anesthetic

Technique
1 Identify the area of interest. If a mass is being resected, the total contour of it and the margins must be taken into account
2 The line and ring blocks are the easiest blocks to perform, as they do not require specific knowledge of neuroanatomy
3 Introduce a long hypodermic needle to its whole length in the subcutaneous tissue
4 Aspirate to prevent accidental intravenous administration and deposit some local anesthetic (e.g. 0.2 mL bupivacaine)
5 Withdraw the needle approximately 5 mm (the distance can vary depending on the volume injected in each point. The bigger the volume, the longer the distance can be), aspirate again and inject a bit more local anesthetic
6 Repeat the sequence until the area of interest is circumscribed
7 When performing ring or curve line blocks, it is recommended to withdraw the needle almost totally before redirecting it in a different direction to prevent tissue damage and needle bending

Cautions
Accidental intravenous injection of local anesthetic. This type of block substitutes for accuracy by using a large volume of local anesthetic. Overdose of local anesthetic is a serious hazard if the total dose is not considered. With this in mind, if the volume is insufficient, use of a more dilute preparation is recommended

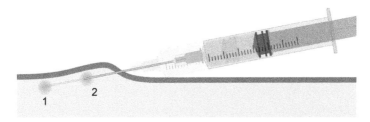

Figure 3.1 Line block. Reproduced with permission from The Ohio State University.

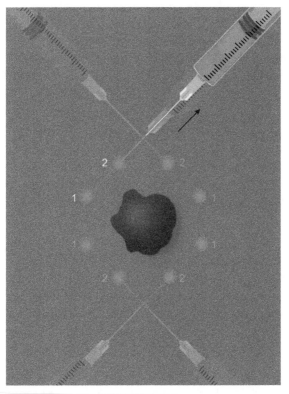

Figure 3.2 Ring block. Performed as a combination of line blocks to avoid needle bending. Reproduced with permission from The Ohio State University.

Inverted "L" block

Indications
Surgical resection of cutaneous or superficial masses, surgical closure of lacerations

Target nerves
Cutaneous nerves originating in the dorsal spinal nerves

Region anesthetized
The area of interest usually is located within the trunk of the animal. Classically, this technique has been used to desensitize the flank

Landmarks
Surrounding tissue around the area of interest. It is fundamental to identify the subcutaneous tissue and the muscular layers, if there is an involvement of these structures

Needle
Hypodermic needle. It is recommended to use a longer length but small in size needle (e.g. 23 Ga 2.5–3.8 cm)

Depth
Subcutaneous injection of local anesthetic

Technique
1 Identify the area of interest. If a mass is being resected, the total contour of it and the margins must be taken into account
2 Following the steps described in the previous block, two line blocks must be performed (forming the inverted "L")
3 Perform a line block between the mass (or area of interest) and the patient's spine
4 Add another line block cranial to the area of interest
5 If there is involvement of muscular layers, it is necessary to block the subcutaneous tissue (for blocking the cutaneous branches of the nerves), but also to perform a deep block to block the muscular branches. The injection of local anesthetic in the muscle is very stimulating, so the subcutaneous block is advisable before attempting the deeper block

Cautions
Accidental intravenous injection of local anesthetic. Overdose of local anesthetic is a serious hazard as a great volume of local anesthetic may be necessary to desensitize a large area of the body. Dilution of the local anesthetic with sterile saline may be an option to achieve the desired volume

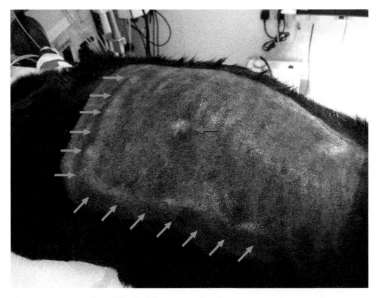

Figure 3.3 Inverted "L" block (*blue arrows*) for the resection of mast cell tumor (*red arrow*).

Block of the surgical incision

This block can be achieved by a single injection at the time of closure or via a diffusion catheter placed in the deep layers of the surgical incision allowing continuous administration of local anesthetics.

Single injection of the surgical incision

Indications
Analgesia of wounds or surgical incisions

Target nerves
Cutaneous nerves of the affected area

Region anesthetized
Surgical incision edges

Landmarks
Subcutaneous tissue around the incision

Needle
23–25 Ga 1.6–1.9 cm hypodermic needle

Depth
Skin to subcutaneous tissue

Technique
1 Probably the oldest and easiest nerve block to perform
2 The injection of local anesthetic in the subcutaneous tissue exposed in the surgical wound is more effective than a simple splash of the drug in the incision
3 Injection of local anesthetic should be done in the same way as the line block (see previous description in this chapter)

    Savvas et al (2008) reported better results when the block was performed before the first incision than when it was performed before suturing.

Cautions
Overdose of local anesthetic is a serious hazard as a great volume of local anesthetic may be necessary to desensitize a large area of the body. Dilution of the local anesthetic with sterile saline may be an option to achieve the desired volume

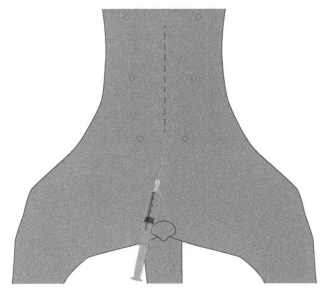

Figure 3.4 Single injection incisional block. Reproduced with permission from The Ohio State University.

Diffusion catheter/"soaker" catheter/"pain buster"

Indications
Analgesia of wounds or surgical incisions

Target nerves
Cutaneous nerves of the affected area

Region anesthetized
Surgical incision from deep layers to skin edges

Landmarks
Surgical incision

Needle
None. The catheter is a flexible polyurethane tube of small diameter with multiple pores for even distribution of the local anesthetic. The catheter is placed during the surgical closure of the incision

Depth
Skin to the deepest layers of the surgical wound

Technique
1 Using a pair of artery forceps and a scalpel, introduce the catheter a few centimeters from the incision edge (so it does not interfere with healing)
2 Place the catheter in the deeper layers of the incision
3 Make sure the length of tube with pores is completely in the incision and that it is long enough for the size of the incision
4 Close the soft tissue above the catheter
5 Secure the catheter externally to the skin to prevent its movement
6 The analgesia can be achieved by the intermittent administration of bupivacaine 2 mg/kg every 6 h (some overlapping between administrations is required as local anesthetics can sting during administration). A constant infusion avoids an analgesia "gap" between doses. Constant infusion dose of lidocaine: dogs 2–3 mg/kg/h, cats 1–1.5 mg/kg/h

Hansen et al (2013) demonstrated no difference between commercial catheters and handmade ones. They also found that very slow infusion rates produce an erratic distribution of the drug.

Cautions
The total volume to be used is dependent on the incision length and not the size of the patient. Always double-check the total dose to be injected and dilute it with sterile saline, if the volume is not sufficient.

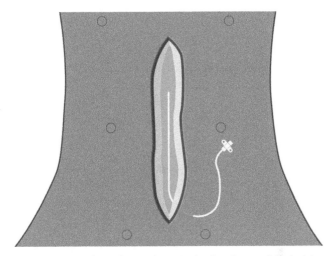

Figure 3.5 Placement of a soaking catheter in the deep layers of the incision before closure. Reproduced with permission from The Ohio State University.

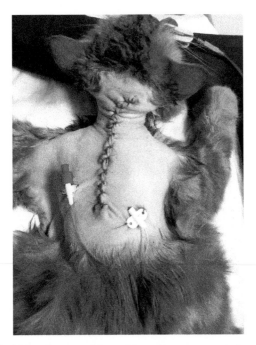

Figure 3.6 Soaking catheter used in a cat for pain management after an injection site sarcoma.

Intercostal blocks

Indications
Lateral thoracotomy, analgesia for rib fractures, analgesia for chest drain placement

Target nerves
Intercostal nerves

Region anesthetized
Intercostal space distal to the injection

Landmarks
Caudal edge of the rib as proximal to the spine as is possible to palpate

Needle
23 Ga 1.9–2.5 cm

Depth
Caudal edge of the rib. *Caution*: introducing the needle further may penetrate the pleura. Directing the tip of the needle underneath the rib may damage the intercostal vein and/or artery

Technique
1 Palpate the caudal edge of the rib and follow it towards the spine
2 Introduce the needle perpendicular to the skin and direct its tip towards the caudal edge of the rib
3 Aspirate to prevent intravascular injection
4 Administer 0.3–1 mL bupivacaine
5 Repeat the previous steps in at least two intercostal spaces cranial and caudal to the area of interest (Thompson & Johnson, 1991). Although desensitizing three spaces, the results are better

  This technique has been shown to be superior to systemic opioids when respiratory function was assessed in patients after lateral thoracotomy (Berg & Orton, 1986).

Cautions
Hematoma, hemothorax, intravascular injection, nerve damage

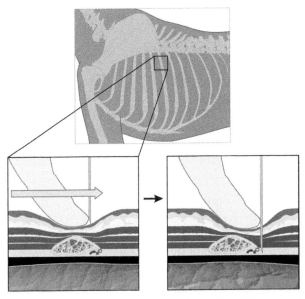

Figure 3.7 Intercostal nerve block. Palpate the rib and then slide the needle over the caudal edge. Reproduced with permission from The Ohio State University.

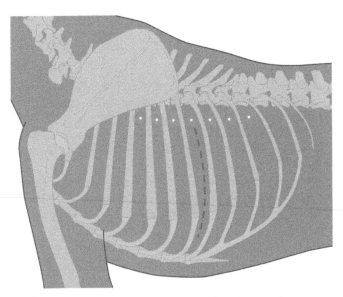

Figure 3.8 An effective intercostal block requires three intercostal spaces on either side of the area of interest. Reproduced with permission from The Ohio State University.

Interpleural block (also known as intrapleural or pleural)

Indications
Classically, this block is indicated for the postoperative management of a lateral thoracotomy or a sternotomy, as it produces less respiratory depression than opioids alone (Berj & Orton, 1986; Conzemius et al, 1994). In human medicine, it is indicated for other conditions, e.g. brachial plexus tumor (Dionne, 1992), cholecystectomy (VadeBoncouer et al, 1989), but veterinary medicine lacks experience in these uses.

Target nerves
The mechanism of action is unknown. It is speculated that the technique may work at three levels: intercostal nerves (due to a retrograde diffusion though the parietal pleura), blockage of the sympathetic chain and the splanchnic nerves, and/or blockage of the ipsilateral brachial plexus.

Region anesthetized
Thoracic cavity, cranial abdominal cavity

Landmarks
Interpleural cavity in an intercostal space

Needle
Over-the-needle catheter (14–18 Ga 4.8–3.2 cm)

Depth
Skin to interpleural cavity

Technique
For repeatable block, it is advisable to place an indwelling thoracic drain or diffusion catheter although the technique may be performed by single injection.

1 Introduce the catheter through the skin over an intercostal space and advance the tip of the needle, tunneling in the subcutaneous tissue to the following intercostal space
2 Penetrate the thoracic wall at the intercostal space, avoiding the caudal edge of the rib where the nerve, artery, and vein are located
3 Introduce the catheter at a shallow angle to decrease the chance of damaging the lung
4 Analgesia can be provided with bupivacaine 2 mg/kg every 5–6 h

Cautions
Pneumothorax, hemothorax, overdose of local anesthetic. Complications are rare if the catheter/chest drain is manipulated carefully. The cardiopulmonary effects of the local anesthetics in the interpleural space are very transient and not clinically significant, even after pericardectomy (Bernard et al, 2006)

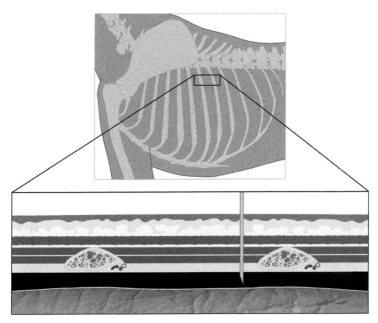

Figure 3.9 Interpleural block. The needle is introduced closer to the cranial edge of the rib to avoid the intercostal vessels. Reproduced with permission from The Ohio State University.

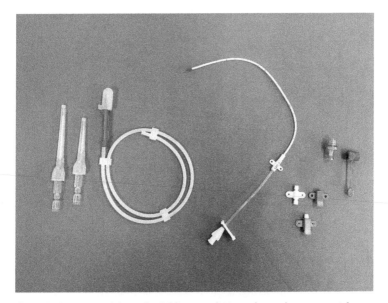

Figure 3.10 Commercial set of a Seldinger technique chest tube commercial. From left to right: over-the-needle catheters for wire insertion, metallic guide-wire, chest tube, holding butterflies, and one-way valve.

Intraperitoneal block

Indications
Analgesia of the abdominal cavity. This block has become a common postoperative analgesic technique for laparotomies and laparoscopies in human medicine

Target nerves
Splanchnic nerves responsible for the visceral component of the abdominal pain

Region anesthetized
Abdominal cavity (exclusively the visceral component)

Landmarks
Abdominal cavity (specifically the area of interest, e.g. ovary, kidney, gallbladder …)

Needle
No needle is required, it is applied in the abdomen before closing the linea alba

Depth
Abdominal cavity

Technique
1 Use 1–2 mg/kg bupivacaine
2 Dilute with sterile saline if the area of interest is too large for the calculated volume
3 Splash the local anesthetic over the area of interest, for instance the ovarian pedicle
4 Alternatively, splash the volume into the cavity, trying to achieve a uniform distribution
5 Close linea alba
  Some authors recommend infiltration of the surgical incision to minimize parietal or somatic pain (Carpenter et al, 2004).

Cautions
The total volume to be used is dependent on the abdominal cavity or the size of the area of interest and not so much on the length and size of the patient. Always double-check the total dose to be injected and dilute it with sterile saline, if the volume is not sufficient.

References

Berg, R.J. & Orton, E.C. (1986) Pulmonary function in dogs after intercostal thoracotomy: comparison of morphine, oxymorphone, and selective intercostal nerve block. *Am J Vet Res* **47**: 471–474.

Bernard, F., Kudnig, S.T. & Monnet, E. (2006) Hemodynamic effects of interpleural lidocaine and bupivacaine combination in anesthetized dogs with and without and open pericardium. *Vet Surg* **35**: 252–258.

Carpenter, R.E., Wilson, D.V. & Evans, A.T. (2004) Evaluation of intraperitoneal and incisional lidocaine or bupivacaine for analgesia following ovariohysterectomy in the dog. *Vet Anaesth Analg* **31**: 46–52.

Conzemius, M.G., Brockman, D.J., King, L.G., et al. (1994) Analgesia in dogs after intercostals thoracotomy: clinical trial comparing intravenous buprenorphine and interpleural bupivacaine. *Vet Surg* **23**: 291–298.

Dionne, C. (1992) Tumour invasion of the brachial plexus: management of pain with interplural analgesia. *Can J Anaesth* **39**: 520–521.

Hansen, B., Lascelles, B.D., Thomson, A., et al. (2013) Variability of performance of wound infusion catheters. *Vet Anaesth Analg* **40**(3): 308–315.

Savvas, I., Papazoglou, L.G., Kazakos, G., et al. (2008) Incisional block with bupivacaine for analgesia after celiotomy in dogs. *J Am Anim Hosp Assoc* **44**(2): 60–66.

Thompson, S.E. & Johnson, J.M. (1991) Analgesia in dogs after intercostal thoracotomy. A comparison of morphine, selective intercostals nerve block, and interpleural regional analgesia with bupivacaine. *Vet Surg* **20**: 73–77.

VadeBoncouer, T.R., Riegler, F.X., Gautt, R.S., et al. (1989) A randomized, double blind comparison of the effects of interpleural bupivacaine and saline on morphine requirements and pulmonary function after cholecystectomy. *Anesthesiology* 71: 339–343.

CHAPTER 4

Blocks of the Head

Fernando Martinez Taboada

Handbook of Small Animal Regional Anesthesia and Analgesia Techniques, First Edition.
By Phillip Lerche, Turi K. Aarnes, Gwen Covey-Crump and Fernando Martinez Taboada.
© 2016 John Wiley & Sons, Ltd. Published 2016 by John Wiley & Sons, Ltd.

Retrobulbar

Indications
Surgical procedures involving the eye and/or procedures requiring akinesia of the eye

Target nerves
Ophthalmic division of the trigeminal nerve (V) (sensory perception), also within the ocular cone, cranial nerves optic (II), oculomotor (III) and abducens (VI) (motor function of the extraocular muscles). The trochlear nerve (IV) is outside the ocular cone, but is frequently blocked by diffusion of the anesthetic drugs and contributes to the akinesia of the eye

Region anesthetized
Eye including conjunctiva, cornea, and uvea

Landmarks
Eye globe, orbit of the eye, zygomatic arch, vertical ramus of the mandible

Needle
22 Ga 2.5 cm (up to 3.8 cm, depending on animal size)

Depth
Skin to ocular cone

Technique
1 Locate the depression limited by the caudal aspect of the maxilla, the ventral edge of the zygomatic arch and the vertical ramus of the mandible
2 Introduce the needle perpendicular to the long axis of the head
3 As soon as the needle tip is in the subcutaneous tissue, direct the needle mediodorsal (behind the zygomatic arch) towards the ocular cone
4 Accurate location of the tip of the needle can be confirmed as the pressure of the needle against the extraocular muscles produce a ventrodorsal movement of the globe
5 Aspirate to prevent intravascular injection
6 Inject 1–2 mL of anesthetic solution or combination (e.g. 0.25–0.5% bupivacaine)

Cautions
Hematoma, intravascular injection, nerve damage. Intraocular damage is rare, although intraconal hematomas can cause blindness. The traditional approach for this block, curving a spinal needle (20 Ga 7.5 cm), has been associated with failure of the technique and risk of direct subarachnoid injection. For this reason, this alternative approach is presented here, although further research comparing differences in safety is still needed

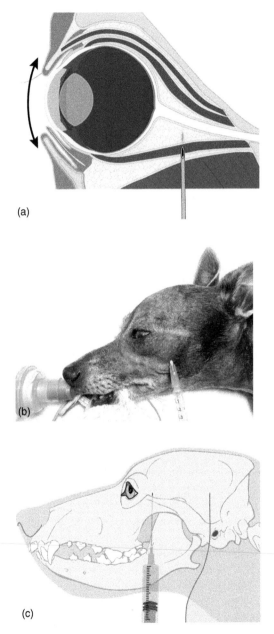

(a)

(b)

(c)

Figure 4.1 (a) Insertion of the needle in the ocular cone produces ventrodorsal movement of the globe. (b–c) Retrobulbar block (subzygomatic approach). Parts (a) and (c) reproduced with permission from The Ohio State University.

Maxillary

Indications
Surgical procedures involving the maxilla, upper lip and/or palate, dental extractions (Aguiar et al, 2015) and rhinoscopy (if performed bilaterally) (Cremer et al, 2013)

Target nerves
Maxillary nerve (ideally with its branches: the nasal and major palatine nerves)

Region anesthetized
Dorsal head and muzzle approximately up to midline. Maxilla and maxillary teeth, hard and soft palate (if major palatine nerve is blocked with the technique), nares, upper labium and rostral part of the nasal cavity

Landmarks
Zygomatic arch, caudal part of the maxilla, and vertical ramus of the mandible

Needle
22 Ga 2.5 cm non-insulated needle

Depth
Skin to pterygoid fossa

Technique
1 Identify the depression formed by the caudal aspect of the maxilla, the ventral edge of the zygomatic arch, and vertical ramus of the mandible. This depression is located ventral to the lateral canthus of the eye
2 Introduce the needle perpendicular to the maxilla
3 Direct the tip of the needle perpendicular to the sagittal plane of the skull
4 If the tip of the needle hits bone, withdraw approximately 1–2 mm before performing the injection
5 Aspirate to prevent intravascular injection
6 Inject 0.3–1 mL of anesthetic solution or combination (e.g. 0.25–0.5% bupivacaine or ropivacaine)

Cautions
Hematoma, intravascular injection, nerve damage

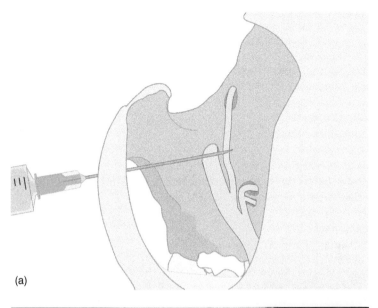

(a)

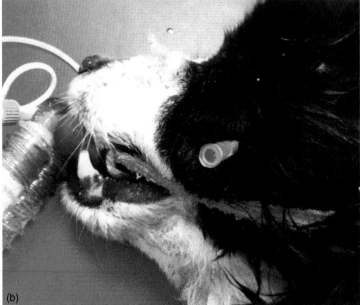

(b)

Figure 4.2 (a) Maxillary nerve block. Needle is directed perpendicular to the pterygoid fossa to also block the nasal and palatal nerve branches. (b) Maxillary nerve block. Part (a) reproduced with permission from The Ohio State University.

Infraorbital

Indications
Surgical procedures involving the rostral part of the muzzle (some procedures may require bilateral block)

Target nerves
Infraorbital nerve

Region anesthetized
Rostral part of the muzzle including skin, maxilla, maxillary teeth, and palate. Rostral upper lip and nasal cavity

Landmarks
Infraorbital foramen, premolar tooth P3

Needle
25 Ga 1.5 or 2.5 cm hypodermic needle

Depth
Skin to the interior of the infraorbital foramen

Technique
1 Percutaneously or lifting the upper lip, locate the infraorbital foramen (dorsal to the tooth P3)
2 Introduce the needle at a shallow angle towards the entrance of the foramen
3 Advance the needle into the foramen as far as possible (within a safety margin, a few millimetres is sufficient)
4 Aspirate to avoid intravascular injection
5 Inject 0.3–0.5 mL of anesthetic solution or combination (e.g. 0.25–0.5% bupivacaine)
6 The effectiveness of the block and the size of the area desensitized depend on whether the injection is performed inside the foramen (anesthetizing up to the first molar; Gross et al, 1997) or only at the entrance (blocking only the area rostral to the canine teeth)

Cautions
Hematoma, intravascular injection, nerve damage

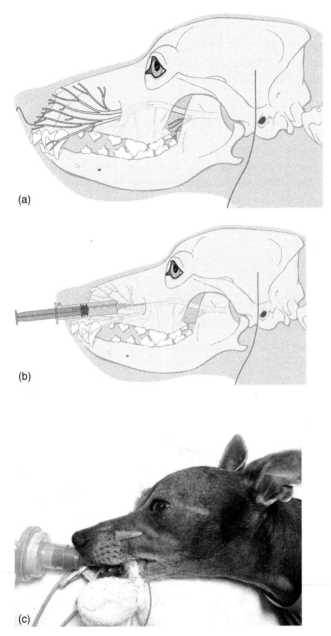

Figure 4.3 (a) Nerve branches exiting the infraorbital foramen. (b) Infraorbital block (note the insertion of the needle tip within the canal). (c) Infraorbital block. Parts (a) and (b) reproduced with permission from The Ohio State University.

Mandibular (or inferior alveolar)

Indications
Surgical procedures involving the mandible, lower lip, and dental extractions (Aguiar et al, 2015)

Target nerves
Inferior alveolar nerve (at the mandibular foramen)

Region anesthetized
Hemi-mandible up to the chin. The tissues between the mandibles should not be anesthetized if the technique is performed correctly. On some occasions, the most rostral part of the chin is not desensitized (in some animals the innervation is by the mylohyoid nerve)

Landmarks
Mandible, angular process, mandibular foramen

Needle
22 Ga 1.6 or 2.5 cm

Depth
Skin rostral to the angular process of the mandible to the mandibular foramen

Technique
1 Palpate the angular process of the mandible, then open the mouth and palpate the mandibular foramen. This foramen is located approximately halfway between the last molar tooth and the condylar process
2 Introduce the needle percutaneously immediately rostral to the angular process and directed dorsally along the medial aspect of the mandible
3 Direct the tip of the needle towards the foramen. It is very difficult to advance the needle into the foramen, but the block can be effective as long as the anesthetic solution is delivered at the entrance of the foramen
4 Aspirate to prevent intravascular injection
5 Inject 0.2–1 mL of anesthetic solution or combination (e.g. 0.25–0.5% bupivacaine)

Cautions
Hematoma, intravascular injection, nerve damage. Desensitization of the tongue can occur if a bilateral block is performed with large volumes and/or poor technique (difficulty locating and injecting within the foramen or as close as possible to it). This desensitization may lead to self-mutilation of the tongue

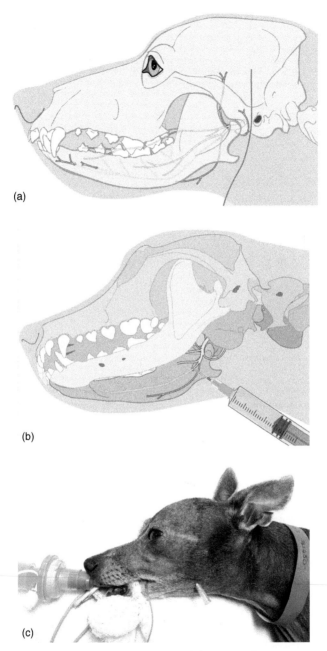

(a)

(b)

(c)

Figure 4.4 (a) Innervation of the mandible and the tongue. (b) Percutaneous approach to the mandibular nerve (note the needle tip close to the foramen). (c) Percutaneous approach for the mandibular nerve block. Parts (a) and (b) reproduced with permission from The Ohio State University.

Mental (or middle mental)

Indications
Surgical procedures involving the rostral mandible, teeth associated with the area, and rostral lower lip

Target nerves
Inferior alveolar (at the mental foramen; also known as the mental nerve)

Region anesthetized
Chin when performed bilaterally, up to premolar tooth P4 if injection is performed inside the foramen (Gross et al, 2000)

Landmarks
Mental foramen, lower lip, premolar tooth P2

Needle
25 Ga 1.6 mm

Depth
Gum mucosa to foramen

Technique
1 Palpate the foramen ventral to the tooth P2 from the inside of the lower lip
2 Introduce the needle just rostral to that point, at a shallow angle, towards the foramen
3 Advance the needle into the foramen as far as possible (without forcing it in)
4 Aspirate to prevent intravascular injection
5 Inject 0.2–0.6 mL of anesthetic solution or combination (e.g. 0.25–0.5% bupivacaine)

Cautions
Hematoma, intravascular injection, nerve damage. In some instances, the most rostral part of the chin is not desensitized (in some animals the innervation is by the mylohyoid nerve)

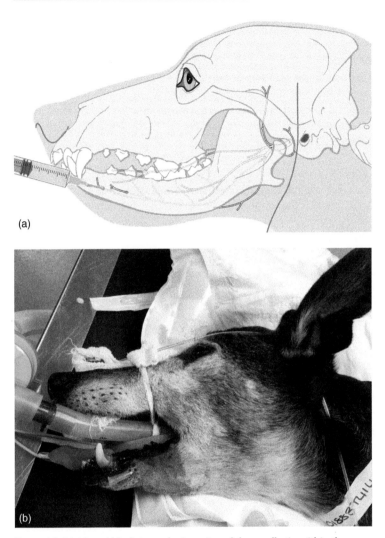

(a)

(b)

Figure 4.5 (a) Mental block (note the insertion of the needle tip within the nerve canal). (b) Mental block for rostral hemimandibulectomy. Part (a) reproduced with permission from The Ohio State University.

Auriculotemporal and great auricular

Indications
Analgesia in severe cases of otitis externa, perioperative analgesia for surgical interventions affecting the external ear canal and the auricular pinna (postoperative analgesia can also be achieved by local infiltration at the time of closure, but the use of this block would provide intraoperative analgesia as well)

Target nerves
Auriculotemporal (branch of the mandibular nerve) and great auricular (formed by the union of the ventral roots of C1 and C2)

Region anesthetized
External ear canal and pinna

Landmarks
Zygomatic arch, external ear canal, vertebral atlas transverse process (also known as wings)

Needle
22 Ga 2.5 cm (or longer in big dogs)

Depth
Skin to mid-distance between skin and temporomandibular joint (auriculotemporal nerve) and skin to subcutaneous tissue (great auricular nerve)

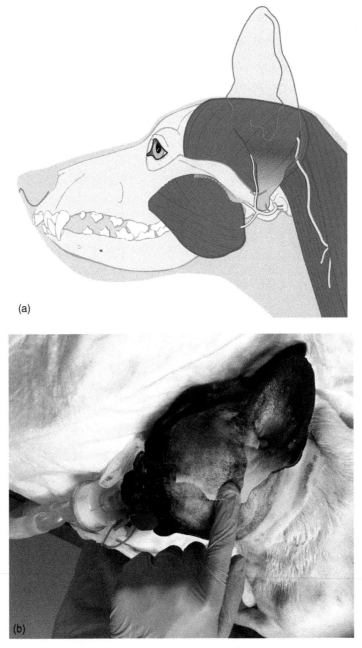

Figure 4.6 (a) Innervation of the ear and pinna. (b) Identification of the anatomical landmarks for the desensitization of the auriculotemporal nerve.

Technique

Auriculotemporal nerve block
1 Palpate the external ear canal (it is conical in shape and very hard when inflamed)
2 Locate the caudal aspect of the zygomatic arch
3 Introduce the needle perpendicular to the skin in the palpable depression between the zygomatic arch and the external ear canal
4 Advance the needle as far as possible until the tip is touching bone (the temporomandibular joint)
5 Knowing the total depth of the tissues, withdraw the needle approximately halfway
6 Aspirate to prevent intravascular injection
7 Inject 0.5–1.5 mL of anesthetic solution or combination (e.g. 0.25–0.5% bupivacaine)

Great auricular nerve
1 Palpate the external ear canal
2 Locate the most cranial point of the transverse process of the atlas vertebra
3 Introduce the needle parallel to the transverse process
4 Direct the tip of the needle ventral to the most cranial part of the process
5 The nerve is very superficial and it is better to maintain the needle at a very shallow angle to the skin
6 Aspirate to prevent intravascular injection
7 Inject 0.5–1.5 mL of anesthetic solution or combination (e.g. 0.25–0.5% bupivacaine)

Cautions
Hematoma, intravascular injection, nerve damage. Temporary paralysis of the facial and/or temporopalpebral nerves preventing the animal from blinking (recommended to lubricate the eye every 2–4 h)

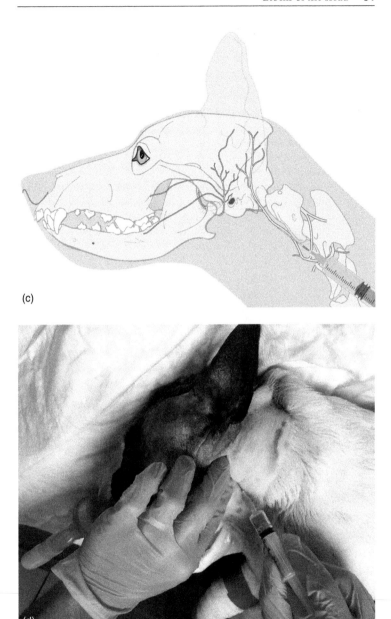

Figure 4.6 (continued)
(c) Innervation in relation to anatomical landmarks. (d) Great auricular nerve block. Parts (a) and (c) reproduced with permission from The Ohio State University.

References

Aguiar, J., Chebroux, A., Martinez-Taboada, F., et al. (2015) Analgesic effects of maxillary and inferior alveolar nerve blocks in cats undergoing dental extractions. *J Feline Med Surg* **17**: 110–116.

Cremer, J., Sum, S.O., Braun, C., et al. (2013) Assessment of maxillary and infraorbital nerve blockade for rhinoscopy in sevoflurane anesthetized dogs. *Vet Anaesth Analg* **40**: 432–439.

Gross, M.E., Pope, E.R., O'Brien, D., et al. (1997) Regional anesthesia of the infraorbital and inferior alveolar nerves during noninvasive tooth pulp stimulation in halothane-anesthetized dogs. *J Am Vet Med Assoc* **211**: 1403–1405.

Gross, M.E., Pope, E.R., Jarboe, J.M., et al. (2000) Regional anesthesia of the infraorbital and inferior alveolar nerves during noninvasive tooth pulp stimulation in halothane-anesthetized cats. *Am J Vet Res* **61**: 1245–1247.

CHAPTER 5

Regional Anesthetic Blocks of the Limbs

Gwen Covey-Crump

Handbook of Small Animal Regional Anesthesia and Analgesia Techniques, First Edition.
By Phillip Lerche, Turi K. Aarnes, Gwen Covey-Crump and Fernando Martinez Taboada.
© 2016 John Wiley & Sons, Ltd. Published 2016 by John Wiley & Sons, Ltd.

Thoracic limb regional anesthetic blocks

Table 5.1 Elicited motor responses to nerve stimulation – thoracic limb

Technique	Motor response	Muscle	Nerves	Accept	Comment
Cervical paravertebral	Hiccup	Diaphragm	Phrenic	✗	Too ventral/caudal
	Adduct, rotate scapula/shoulder	Supraspinatus, infraspinatus	Suprascapular	✗✓	Cranial
			Subscapular		
brachial plexus	Rotate shoulder in, flex elbow	Biceps brachialis	Musculocutaneous	✓	Cranial aspect of technique
	Flex shoulder, extend elbow/carpus	Teres major/minor, deltoideus	Axillary	✓	Middle aspect of technique
	Extend elbow/carpus	Triceps, carpal/digital extensors	Radial	✓✓	Local anesthetic here should diffuse over most of brachial plexus
	Pronate antebrachium, carpal/palmar flexion	Carpal/digital flexors	Median	✓	Injection very caudal may not reach more cranial nerves
	Palmar flexion	Carpal/digital flexors	Ulnar	✓	
RUMM	Palmar extension	Carpal/digital extensors	Radial	✓	
	Palmar flexion	Carpal/digital flexors	Median, ulnar	✓	
	Triceps/biceps contraction			✗	Direct muscle stimulation

Brachial plexus

Indications
Unilateral surgical procedures of distal humerus, elbow, antebrachium, carpus

Target nerves
Musculocutaneous, axillary, radial, median and ulnar

Region anesthetized
Thoracic limb distal to mid humerus

Landmarks
Acromion, trachea, jugular vein, 1st rib

Needle
21 Ga 5.0–10.0 cm insulated needle

Depth
Acromion to 1st rib

Technique (Campoy et al, 2008; Mahler & Adogwa, 2008)
1 Identify 1st rib by axillary palpation. Premeasure needle depth to a point where a line extending the course of the jugular vein crosses the 1st rib. The brachial plexus is just cranial to this point
2 Insert needle craniomedial to the acromion in a caudoventral direction parallel to the jugular vein and in a strictly sagittal plane
3 With nerve stimulator at 2 mA and gradually reducing, observe responses to nerve stimulation (Table 5.1) (reducing to 0.2 mA to avoid intrafascicular injection prior to injection)
4 At point of radial nerve stimulation (and no further than premeasured depth), aspirate to avoid intravascular (blood) or interpleural (air) injection
5 Inject 0.1 mL/kg 0.5% bupivacaine or 0.75% ropivacaine
6 Withdraw needle 0.5–1 cm, aspirate, then inject further 0.1 mL/kg
7 Repeat step 6, injecting a final 0.1 mL/kg beneath the point of the shoulder

Cautions
Intravascular, interpleural injection, hematoma. Nerve damage

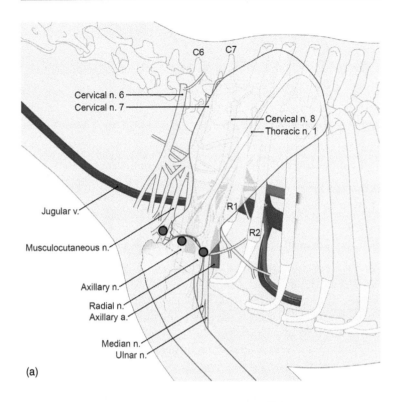

(a)

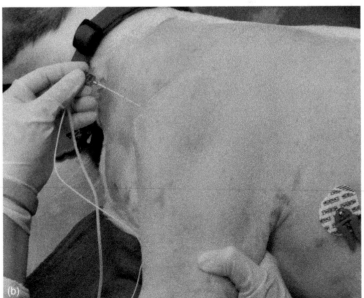

Figure 5.1 Brachial plexus block. (a) Anatomy, (b) approach. Part (a) reproduced with permission from The Ohio State University.

Paravertebral: C6–T1

Indications
Unilateral surgical procedures of the scapula, shoulder, and brachium, including forequarter amputation

Target nerves
Spinal nerves of C6, C7, C8, T1

Region anesthetized
Entire thoracic limb, except skin over upper shoulder region

Landmarks
Transverse process C6, head of rib 1

Needle
21 Ga 5.0 cm insulated (very small dogs) to 15.0 cm (very large dogs)

Technique (Campoy & Read, 2013; Lemke & Creighton, 2008)
Advanced technique to be undertaken with due caution only in patients where palpation of C6 and 1st rib is possible. Unilateral block only

1 With patient in lateral recumbency and limb to be blocked uppermost, retract scapula caudally
2 Palpate transverse process of C6, maintain digital pressure on lateral aspect
3 From dorsolateral approach, advance needle in caudal direction to meet transverse process. Walk needle off cranial border
4 With nerve stimulator at 2 mA and gradually reducing, observe responses to nerve stimulation of ventral branches of spinal nerves C6 and C7, suprascapular, subscapular, musculocutaneous (Table 5.1) (reducing to 0.2 mA to avoid intrafascicular injection prior to injection)
5 Aspirate to avoid intravascular (blood) or spinal (clear fluid) injection
6 Inject 0.1 mL/kg 0.5% bupivacaine or 0.75% ropivacaine
7 Repeat steps 3–6, walking needle off caudal border of transverse process
8 Palpate axillary artery at 1st rib costochondral junction and thoracic inlet. Advance needle to meet cranial aspect 1st rib 1–2 cm dorsal to costochondral junction
9 Observe elbow/carpus/digit extension (C8) and carpus/digit flexion (T1)
10 Aspirate to avoid intravascular (blood) or interpleural (air) injection
11 Inject 0.1 mL/kg 0.5% bupivacaine or 0.75% ropivacaine

Cautions
Intravascular epidural or interpleural injection, hematoma. Nerve injury. Phrenic nerve paralysis (common). Do not perform technique bilaterally

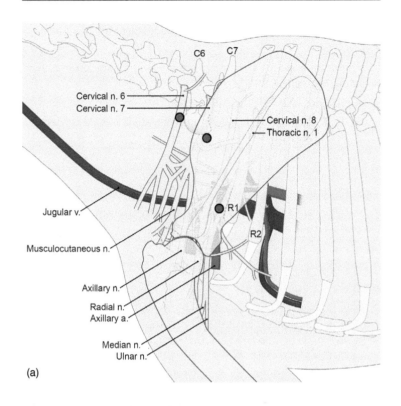

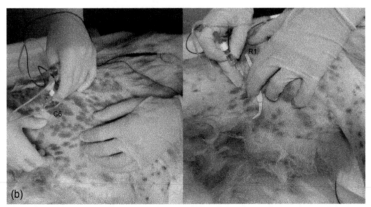

Figure 5.2 Paravertebral block. (a) Anatomy, (b) approach. Part (a) reproduced with permission from The Ohio State University.

RUMM (radial/ulnar/median/musculocutaneous)

Indications
Anesthesia for surgical procedures of the thoracic limb distal to and including the carpus

Target nerves
Radial (R), ulnar (U), median (Me), musculocutaneous (Mus) nerves

Region anesthetized
Carpus, metacarpus, and digits

Landmarks
Lateral and medial epicondyles, greater tubercle of humerus. Lateral and medial head of triceps, biceps and biceps brachialis muscles. Brachial artery

Needle
21 Ga 5.0 cm insulated/20–22 Ga 2.0–4.0 cm non-insulated

Depth
10–20 mm

Technique (Lamont & Lemke, 2008; Trumpatori et al, 2009)
1 Begin with patient in lateral recumbency, limb to treat uppermost, elbow flexed 90°
2 Grasp humerus from cranial aspect, place thumb on caudal humerus two-thirds distance from greater tubercle to lateral epicondyle. Retract brachialis muscle cranially. Insert needle from caudal aspect, perpendicular to long axis of humerus at 45° angle. Puncture long heads of triceps to contact humerus, withdraw slightly
3 If using nerve stimulator, with nerve stimulator at 2 mA and gradually reducing, observe responses to radial nerve stimulation (Table 5.1) (reducing to 0.2 mA to avoid intrafascicular injection prior to injection)
4 Aspirate to avoid intra-arterial injection
5 Inject 0.1 mL/kg 0.5% bupivacaine or 0.75% ropivacaine
6 Turn patient into opposite lateral recumbency, have assistant retract upper limb caudally (limb to treat is lowest and flexed 90°)
7 Palpate brachial artery at point mid humerus. With digital pressure on humerus, retract biceps brachialis muscle and brachial artery cranially. Insert needle from caudal aspect perpendicular to long axis of humerus and at 45° angle to contact humerus, withdraw slightly
8 Observe responses to median/ulnar nerve stimulation if using (Table 5.1)
9 Aspirate to avoid intra-arterial injection
10 Inject half of 0.15 mL/kg 0.5% bupivacaine or 0.75% ropivacaine deeply and remaining half as needle is withdrawn

Cautions
Risk of intravascular injection, nerve damage

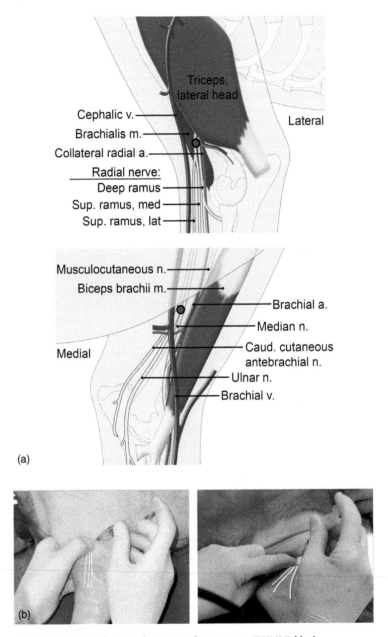

Figure 5.3 Radius, ulnar, median, musculocutaneous (RUMM) block.
(a) Anatomy, (b) approach. Part (a) reproduced with permission from
The Ohio State University.

Bier block (intravenous regional anesthesia) (Staffieri, 2013)

Indications
Surgical procedures of <90 min duration of the distal limb, especially when a bloodless surgical field is advantageous

Target nerves
Local anesthetic effect by spread to peripheral nerve endings

Region anesthetized
Thoracic limb distal to elbow and pelvic limb distal to tarsus

Important anatomy
- Suitable distal vein
- Palpable peripheral artery

Equipment
- Tourniquet – preferably pneumatic with pressure gauge
- Esmarch or elastic bandage
- Doppler probe (optional)
- Catheter 22–25 Ga 25–33 mm

Technique (Webb et al, 1999)
1. Clip surgical and catheter placement sites (plus tourniquet site if heavily coated)
2. Place intravenous catheter as distally as possible
3. Find a palpable artery and mark with pen
4. Apply tourniquet and identify lower occlusion pressure (LOP) (pressure at which palpable pulse is absent)
5. Release tourniquet, apply esmarch or elastic bandage tightly
6. Apply tourniquet to 50–100 mmHg above LOP, record time
7. Release esmarch bandage
8. Confirm absence of peripheral pulse
9. Infuse lidocaine 0.5% 0.6 mL/kg over 2–3 min, observe patient for toxicity
10. Remove catheter
11. During surgery, monitor and maintain cuff pressure 50–100 mmHg above systolic arterial pressure
12. At end of surgery, remove tourniquet slowly, observing for signs of toxicity and to ensure hemostasis

Cautions
Avoid cuff pressures in excess of 400 mmHg. Use only lidocaine. Risk of systemic toxicity, ischemic injury, limb engorgement, tourniquet pain

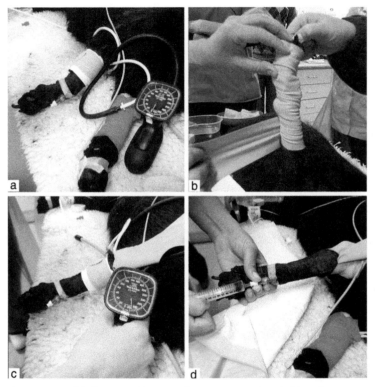

Figure 5.4 Bier block. (a) Find lower occlusion pressure (LOP), (b) apply esmarch bandage, (c) apply tourniquet 50–100 mmHg above LOP and remove esmarch, (d) check pulse absent, infuse lidocaine.

Pelvic limb

Table 5.2 Elicited motor responses to nerve stimulation – pelvic limb

Technique	Motor response	Muscle	Nerves	Accept	Comment
Femoral – inguinal approach	Patellar twitch	Quadriceps	Femoral/ saphenous	✓	
	Anterior thigh	Sartorius		✗	Too superficial
Femoral – lateral preiliac approach (caudal lumbar plexus)	Hip flexion	Psoas stimulation		✗	Direct muscle stimulation
	Hip adduction	Gracilis, pectineus, adductor femoris, obturator externus	Obturator	✗	May block with femoral
	Stifle extension, patellar twitch	Quadriceps	Femoral	✓	
Sciatic – lateral approach	Biceps twitch at 1 mA		Direct muscle stimulation	✗	Too superficial
	Semimembranosus/ tendinosus twitch		Motor branches only	✗	Too caudal
	Stifle flexion	Biceps femoris	Sciatic	✓	
	Plantarflexion	Gastrocnemius	Tibial	✓	
	Dorsiflexion		Peroneal/fibular	✓	
Sciatic – parasacral approach	Gluteal twitch			✗	Direct muscle stimulation
	Stifle flexion	Biceps femoris	Sciatic	✓	
	Plantarflexion	Gastrocnemius	Tibial	✓	
	Dorsiflexion		Peroneal/fibular	✓	

Femoral/saphenous nerve block

Inguinal approach

Indications
Surgery of distal femur, stifle and distal limb in combination with sciatic nerve block

Target nerves
Femoral and/or its branch: saphenous

Region anesthetized
Medial aspect of hindlimb – mid femur to 1st digit

Landmarks
Femoral artery; femoral triangle (enclosed dorsally by rectus femoris, cranially by caudal belly of sartorius muscle, proximally (deep) by iliopsoas muscle

Needle
21 Ga 5.0 cm insulated/20–22 Ga 2.0–4.0 cm non-insulated

Depth
5–15 mm

Technique
1 With patient in lateral recumbency, hindlimb to treat uppermost
2 Abduct limb caudally, palpate femoral artery
3 Direct needle dorsomedially towards nerve which lies cranial to femoral artery
4 With nerve stimulator at 2 mA and gradually reducing, observe responses to nerve stimulation including quadriceps twitch, patellar twitch, stifle extension (Table 5.2) (reducing to 0.2 mA to avoid intrafascicular injection prior to injection) (sartorius twitch = needle too superficial)
5 Aspirate to avoid intra-arterial injection
6 Inject 0.2 mL/kg 0.5% bupivacaine or 0.75% ropivacaine

Cautions
Hematoma, intravascular injection, nerve damage

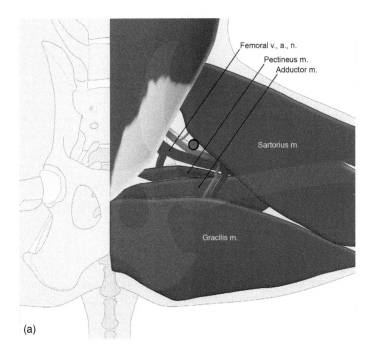

Femoral v., a., n.
Pectineus m.
Adductor m.
Sartorius m.
Gracilis m.

(a)

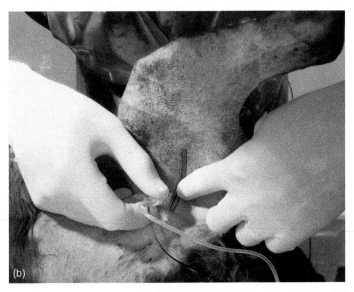

(b)

Figure 5.5 Femoral nerve block – inguinal approach. (a) Anatomy, (b) approach. Part (a) reproduced with permission from The Ohio State University.

Lateral preiliac approach (caudal lumbar plexus) (Portela et al, 2013)

Target nerves
Femoral (may also block obturator)

Region anesthetized
Hemipelvis, femur, medial femorotibial joint, skin of dorsomedial tarsus, 1st digit. May not anesthetize skin overlying coxofemoral joint

Landmarks
Cranial dorsal iliac crest (CDIC), L6

Needle
Small dogs 22 Ga 5.0 cm, large dogs 22 Ga 7.5 cm insulated

Depth
Use depth of iliopsoas muscle as reference

Technique
1 With patient in lateral recumbency, hindlimb to treat uppermost
2 Draw a line dorsoventral from L6, bisect with line parallel to spine originating from most cranial aspect of iliac crest
3 Puncture site at bisection, advance needle caudomedially with 30–45° intent through iliocostalis lumborum muscle
4 With nerve stimulator at 1 mA and gradually reducing, observe responses to nerve stimulation – quadriceps contraction (Table 5.2) (reducing to 0.2 mA to avoid intrafascicular injection prior to injection)
5 Aspirate to avoid intra-arterial injection
6 Inject 0.1 mL/kg 0.5% bupivacaine or 0.75% ropivacaine

Cautions
Low risk of epidural migration, vessel puncture

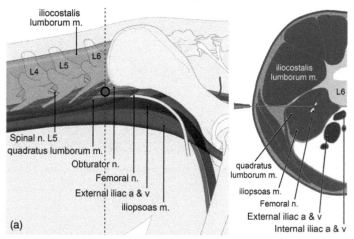

Figure 5.6 (a) Puncture site.

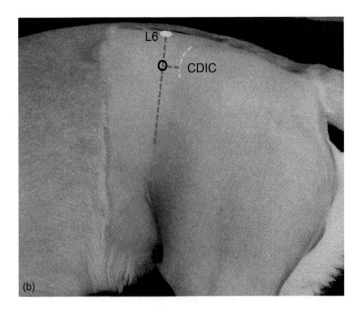

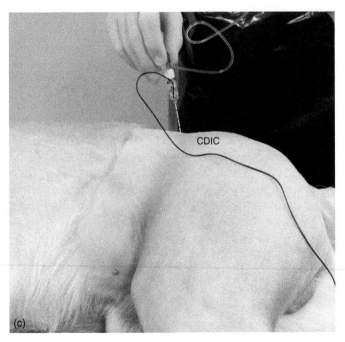

Figure 5.6 Femoral nerve block – lateral preiliac approach. (b) Anatomy, (c) approach. Part (a) reproduced with permission from The Ohio State University.

Sciatic nerve block

Indications
Surgery of distal femur, stifle and distal limb in combination with femoral nerve block

Target nerves
Sciatic (ischiatic) nerve gives off branches: common peroneal, tibial nerves

Region anesthetized
Lateral, dorsal, caudal aspects of hindlimb – caudolateral stifle to digits 2–5

Lateral approach (Campoy et al, 2008)

Landmarks
Greater trochanter of femur (GT), ischial tuberosity (IT)

Needle
21 Ga 5.0 cm insulated or 22 Ga 2.0–4.0 cm non-insulated

Depth
5–10 mm

Technique
1 With patient in lateral recumbency, hindlimb to treat uppermost on a line between GT and IT, puncture site is 1/3 distance from GT
2 Direct needle perpendicular to skin
3 With nerve stimulator at 2 mA and gradually reducing, observe responses to nerve stimulation – dorsiflexion of tarsus (peroneal nerve), plantarflexion (tibial nerve) (Table 5.2) (reducing to 0.2 mA to avoid intrafascicular injection prior to injection)
4 Aspirate to avoid intra-arterial injection
5 Inject 0.05–0.1 mL/kg 0.25–0.5% bupivacaine or 0.75% ropivacaine

Cautions
Risk of intravascular injection, nerve damage

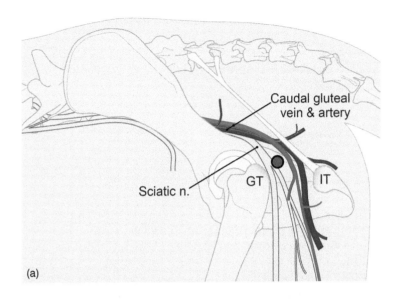

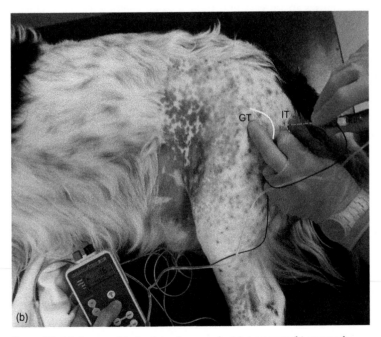

Figure 5.7 Sciatic nerve block – lateral approach. (a) Anatomy, (b) approach. Part (a) reproduced with permission from The Ohio State University.

Parasacral approach (sacral plexus block) (Portela et al, 2010)

Landmarks
Cranial dorsal iliac crest (CDIC), ischial tuberosity (IT), dorsal spinous processes (DSP)

Needle
21 Ga 5.0 cm insulated

Depth
15–30 mm

Technique
1 With patient in lateral recumbency, hindlimb to treat uppermost, on a line between CDIC and IT, puncture site is 1/3 distance from CDIC
2 Direct needle sagitally
3 With nerve stimulator at 2 mA and gradually reducing, observe responses to nerve stimulation – gastrocnemius twitch, digital/tarsal flexion/extension (Table 5.2) (reducing to 0.2 mA to avoid intrafascicular injection prior to injection)
4 Aspirate to avoid intra-arterial injection
5 Inject 0.1 mL/kg 0.5% bupivacaine or 0.75% ropivacaine

Cautions
Risk of intravascular injection, epidural injection, nerve damage, bowel puncture

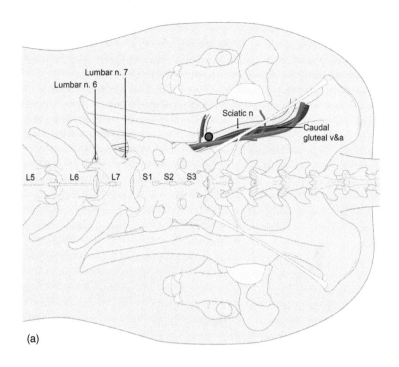

(a)

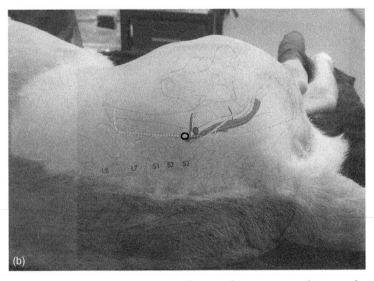

(b)

Figure 5.8 Sciatic nerve block – parasacral approach. (a) Anatomy, (b) approach. Reproduced with permission from The Ohio State University.

References

Campoy, L. & Read, M.R. (2013) The thoracic limb. In: *Small Animal Regional Anesthesia and Analgesia*. Ames, IA: Wiley-Blackwell, pp.146–147.

Campoy, L. Looney, A.L. Ludders, J.W. & Gleed, R.D. (2008) Distribution of a Lidocaine-methylene blue solution staining in brachial plexus, lumbar plexus and sciatic nerve blocks in the dog. *Vet Anaesth Analg* **35**: 348–354.

Lamont, L.A. & Lemke, K.A. (2008) The effects of medetomidine on radial nerve blockade with mepivacaine in dogs. *Vet Anaesth Analg* **35**: 62–68.

Lemke, K.A. & Creighton, C.M. (2008) Paravertebral blockade of the brachial plexus in dogs. *Vet Clin Small Anim* **38**: 1231–1241

Mahler, S.P. & Adogwa, A.O. (2008) Anatomical and experimental studies of brachial plexus, sciatic, and femoral nerve-location using peripheral nerve stimulation in the dog. *Vet Anaesth Analg* **35**: 80–89.

Portela, D.A., Otero, P.E. Tarragona, L., Briganti, A., Breghi, G. & Melanie, P. (2010) Combined paravertebral plexus block and parasacral sciatic block in healthy dogs. *Vet Anaesth Analg* **37**: 531–541.

Portela, D.A., Otero, P.E., Briganti, A., et al. (2013) Femoral nerve block: a novel psoas compartment lateral pre-iliac approach in dogs. *Vet Anaesth Analg* **40**: 194–204.

Staffieri, F. (2013) Intravenous regional anesthesia. In: Campoy, L. & Read, M.R. (eds) *Small Animal Regional Anesthesia and Analgesia*. Ames, IA: Wiley-Blackwell, pp. 261–271.

Trumpatori, B.J., Carter, J.E., Hash, J., et al. (2009) Evaluation of a mid-humeral block of the radial, ulnar, musculocutaneous and median (RUMM block) nerves for analgesia of the distal aspect of the thoracic limb in dogs. *Vet Surg* **39**: 785–796.

Webb, A.A., Cantwell, S.L., Duke, T., et al. (1999) Intravenous regional anesthesia (Bier block) in a dog. *Can Vet J* **40**: 419–421.

CHAPTER 6

Epidurals and Spinals

Turi K. Aarnes

Handbook of Small Animal Regional Anesthesia and Analgesia Techniques, First Edition.
By Phillip Lerche, Turi K. Aarnes, Gwen Covey-Crump and Fernando Martinez Taboada.
© 2016 John Wiley & Sons, Ltd. Published 2016 by John Wiley & Sons, Ltd.

Lumbosacral epidural and spinal in dogs

Indications
Abdominal pain, thoracic pain, hindlimb pain, perineum/tail

Target nerves
Nerves caudal to the spread of local anesthetic

Region of anesthesia/analgesia
Using 0.2 mL/kg of injectate (local anesthetic or morphine at appropriate dose diluted to appropriate volume), anesthesia/analgesia should occur from T13 spinal space and extend caudally. Larger volumes may be used if cranial spread is desired.

Landmarks
Place the thumb and middle finger on the craniodorsal aspects of the wings of the ilium and place the index finger at the lumbosacral space (L7–S1) for epidural administration (Figure 6.1). When performing a spinal, place the thumb and middle finger on the craniodorsal aspects of the wings of the ilium, and the index finger at the space between L5 and L6.

Needle
A spinal needle with stilette (e.g. Tuohy needle for epidural, Quincke needle for spinal), depending on the size of the dog – typically a 20 Ga, 5.1 cm needle for a 15–40 kg dog.

Technique (Skarda & Tranquilli, 2007a; Troncy et al, 2002)
A distinct "pop" is felt when the needle is advanced through the interarcuate ligament (ligamentum flavum) (Figure 6.2). No blood or spinal fluid should be observed when performing an epidural. Fluid will most likely be observed flowing from the needle when the stilette is removed when performing a spinal, though it is possible to be in the subarachnoid space with no fluid flowing ("dry tap"). Loss of resistance technique may be utilized by injecting approximately 1 mL air – no resistance to injection and no backpressure on the syringe plunger should be felt. The "hanging drop technique" may also be used by placing saline into the needle to fill the hub. The drop should be "sucked in" to the epidural space. Minimal or no resistance to injection should be felt during drug administration.

Advantages
Advantages of epidural anesthesia include good muscle relaxation, postoperative analgesia, minimal effects on the body, low cost

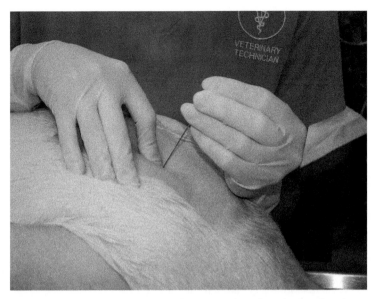

Figure 6.1 Palpation of the lumbosacral space in a dog. Place the thumb and middle finger on the craniodorsal aspects of the wings of the ilium and place the index finger at the lumbosacral space.

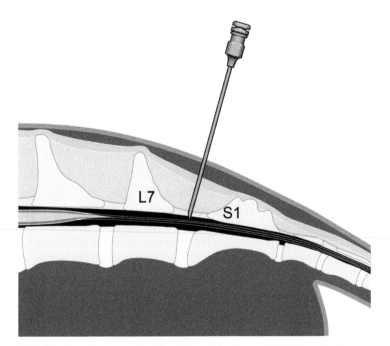

Figure 6.2 Lumbosacral epidural technique in a dog. A distinct "pop" is felt when the needle is advanced through the interarcuate ligament (ligamentum flavum). Reproduced with permission from The Ohio State University.

Complications

Inadequate anesthesia due to faulty technique, if the animal is awake during surgery (might move); hypotension (if using local anesthetic), respiratory depression (local anesthetic epidurals and spinals), or apnea after excessive blockade (epidurals and spinals); accidental administration into the subarachnoid space (if intent is to perform an epidural).

Contraindications

Hypovolemia and hypotension (when using local anesthetics), bleeding disorder, skin infection

Lumbosacral epidural in cats

Indications

Abdominal pain, thoracic pain, hindlimb pain, perineum/tail

Target nerves

Nerves caudal to the spread of local anesthetic

Region of anesthesia/analgesia

Using 0.2 mL/kg of injectate (local anesthetic or morphine at appropriate dose diluted to appropriate volume), anesthesia/analgesia should occur from T13 spinal space and extend caudally. Local anesthetic for lumbosacral epidural should be used with caution in cats due to toxicity/sensitivity and potential for spinal administration.

Landmarks

Place the thumb and middle finger on the craniodorsal aspects of the wings of the ilium and place the index finger at the lumbosacral space (Figure 6.3).

Needle

A 22 Ga 2.5 cm straight needle

Technique (Skarda & Tranquilli, 2007b; Troncy et al, 2002)

A 22 Ga needle is placed at the midline of the lumbosacral space (L7–S1) (Figure 6.4). A distinct "pop" is felt when the needle is advanced through the interarcuate ligament (ligamentum flavum). No blood or spinal fluid should be observed. Minimal resistance to injection should be felt.

Complications

Inadequate anesthesia due to faulty technique, if the animal is awake during surgery (might move); hypotension, respiratory depression, or apnea after excessive blockade; accidental administration into the subarachnoid space. Due to anatomical differences from dogs, more likely to perform a spinal rather than an epidural (spinal cord ends at L6–S2), in which case dose of injected drug should be reduced by 50%.

Contraindications

Hypovolemia and hypotension (when using local anesthetics), bleeding disorder, skin infection. Reduce dose by 50% if performing spinal rather than epidural.

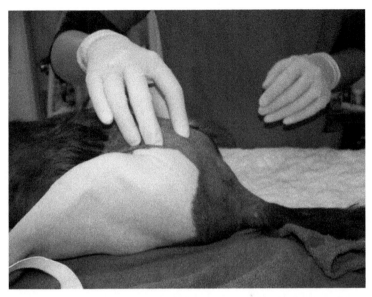

Figure 6.3 Palpation of the lumbosacral space in a cat. Place the thumb and middle finger on the craniodorsal aspects of the wings of the ilium and place the index finger at the lumbosacral space.

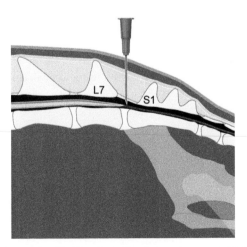

Figure 6.4 Lumbosacral epidural and spinal technique in a cat. A 22 Ga needle is placed at the midline of the lumbosacral (L7–S1) space. Reproduced with permission from The Ohio State University.

Caudal epidural in dogs and cats

Indications
Described for use in cats with urethral obstruction. Other possibilities: dystocia, tail amputation, perineal procedures

Target nerves
Nerves caudal to the spread of local anesthetic

Region of anesthesia/analgesia
Perineum, tail, sacrum

Landmarks
A coccygeal epidural can be performed at either the sacrococcygeal interspace or Co1–Co2. First moveable vertebrae between the sacrum and tail, or first coccygeal interspace, on midline

Needle
25 Ga 1.5 cm straight needle

Technique (O'Hearn & Wright, 2011)
Palpate the space between sacrum and Co1 or Co1 and Co2. Insert 25 Ga needle on midline, direct at a 30–45° angle, and advance through the ligamentum flavum (Figure 6.5). Aspirate through the needle to check for blood (if blood is aspirated, start over). Infuse 0.1–0.2 mL/kg of lidocaine 2%.

Complications
Bleeding, incomplete blockade

Contraindications
Hypovolemia and hypotension (when using local anesthetics), bleeding disorder, skin infection

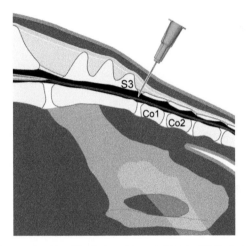

Figure 6.5 Coccygeal epidural technique in a cat. Insert a 25 Ga needle on the midline, directed at a 30–45° angle, and advance through the ligamentum flavum. Reproduced with permission from The Ohio State University.

References

O'Hearn, A.K. & Wright, B.D. (2011) Coccygeal epidural with local anesthetic for catherization and pain management in the treatment of feline urethral obstruction. *J Vet Emerg Crit Care* **21**: 50–52.

Skarda, R.T. & Tranquilli, W.J. (2007a) Local and regional anesthetic and analgesic techniques: dogs. In: Tranquilli, W.J., Thurmon, J.C. & Grimm, K.A. (eds) *Lumb & Jones' Veterinary Anesthesia and Analgesia*, 4th edn. Ames, IA: Wiley-Blackwell, pp.561–594.

Skarda, R.T. & Tranquilli, W.J. (2007b) Local and regional anesthetic and analgesic techniques: cats. In: Tranquilli, W.J., Thurmon, J.C. & Grimm, K.A. (eds) *Lumb & Jones' Veterinary Anesthesia and Analgesia*, 4th edn. Ames, IA: Wiley-Blackwell, pp.595-603.

Troncy, E., Junot, S., Keroack, S., et al. (2002) Results of preemptive epidural administration of morphine with or without bupivacaine in dogs and cats undergoing surgery: 265 cases (1997–1999). *J Am Vet Med Assoc* **221**: 666–672.

CHAPTER 7

Emergency Procedures

Turi K. Aarnes

Handbook of Small Animal Regional Anesthesia and Analgesia Techniques, First Edition.
By Phillip Lerche, Turi K. Aarnes, Gwen Covey-Crump and Fernando Martinez Taboada.
© 2016 John Wiley & Sons, Ltd. Published 2016 by John Wiley & Sons, Ltd.

Complications associated with local anesthetic techniques

Bleeding

Bleeding is a potential complication of all nerve blocks. Caution should be exercised in patients with bleeding/clotting disorders and patients that have been heparinized. Epidurals and spinals are contraindicated in these patients.

Clinical signs
Visible hemorrhage, hypotension

Treatment
Monitor systemic blood pressure, apply pressure to area of hemorrhage, cold compress to reduce blood flow, in extreme cases ligation of blood vessels (e.g. accidental laceration of an artery)

Nerve trauma

Injection of local anesthetic directly into nerve or nerve trauma may result from local anesthetic techniques. Return to normal function may occur over time.

Clinical signs
Pain, motor or sensory deficits, urinary or fecal incontinence

Treatment
Supportive care, systemic analgesics for pain, systemic anti-inflammatories

Complications associated with local anesthetic drugs

Allergic reactions to local anesthetic drugs

True allergic reactions to local anesthetics are rare. Reported with use of aminoesters (e.g. procaine, tetracaine). Signs develop 12–24 h after exposure (Lin & Liu, 2013).

Clinical signs
Hypersensitivity reaction; contact dermatitis including erythema, pruritus, papules, vesicles

Treatment
Stop administration of local anesthetic, airway maintenance, epinephrine, intravenous fluids, diphenhydramine

Methemoglobinemia
More likely with benzocaine or prilocaine but also reported with procaine and lidocaine. Also more likely in cats than dogs.

Clinical signs
Hypoxia, cyanosis, death, blood that looks brown in color, dyspnea, nausea, tachycardia

Treatment
Intravenous administration of 1% methylene blue; intubation and oxygen supplementation, ventilation, ECG monitoring (Stoelting & Hillier, 2006).

Systemic toxicity of local anesthetics
Systemic toxicity of local anesthetics is usually associated with increased plasma concentrations. Systemic toxicities may result in cardiac arrest. Monitoring patients and preparation for performing CPCR are necessary.

Cardiovascular toxicity (Table 7.1)
Cardiovascular (CV) toxicity is increased with bupivacaine compared with lidocaine or ropivacaine, accidental intravenous administration of bupivacaine or ropivacaine, and in patients with decreased hepatic function. Large doses of high-potency local anesthetics are more likely to result in CV toxicity leading to complete AV block and CV collapse. Separately, CV toxicity may result from CNS toxicity due to decreased activity of the nucleus tractus solitarii resulting in decreased autonomic control of the CV system (Salinas et al, 2004).

CNS toxicity (Table 7.2)
Related to plasma concentration and potency. Low concentrations cause CNS depression, high concentrations can result in excitation due to inhibition of inhibitory neurons. High potency and high lipid solubility can result in increased CNS toxicity (Lin & Liu, 2013).

Table 7.1 Cardiovascular toxicity

Complication	Mechanism	Clinical presentation/clinical sign	Treatment
Vasodilation	Excessive plasma concentration, also related to potency of local anesthetic drug	Hypotension, collapse, tachycardia	Stop administration of local anesthetic, continuous monitoring of invasive blood pressure, administer IV fluids, vasopressors (vasopressin, epinephrine, ephedrine, phenylephrine), inotropes (dopamine, dobutamine), intravenous lipid emulsion
Dysrhythmias	Excessive plasma concentration, unbound drug diffuses to conducting tissue of heart, also related to potency of local anesthetic drug	ECG changes: prolongation of P-R interval, prolongation of QRS interval, AV block, ventricular premature contractions, ventricular tachycardia, ventricular fibrillation	Stop administration of local anesthetic, continuous monitoring of ECG, intravenous lipid emulsion, antidysrhythmics, oxygen supplementation
Myocardial depression and cardiac toxicity	Unbound drug diffuses to conducting tissue of heart, inhibition of depolarization rate of cardiac action potential due to sodium channel blockade; most likely with accidental IV administration of bupivacaine Epinephrine and phenylephrine may increase bupivacaine toxicity to cAMP inhibition	ECG changes, hypotension	Stop administration of local anesthetic, continuous monitoring of invasive blood pressure, continuous ECG monitoring, intravenous fluids, administer IV fluids, vasopressors (vasopressin, epinephrine, ephedrine, phenylephrine), inotropes (dopamine, dobutamine), intravenous lipid emulsion (Weinberg et al, 2003), antidysrhythmics, oxygen supplementation

Table 7.2 CNS toxicity

Complication	Mechanism	Clinical presentation/clinical sign	Treatment
CNS depression/toxicity	Excessive plasma concentration (dose dependent), also related to potency of local anesthetic drug	Nystagmus, myoclonus, seizures	Stop administration of local anesthetic, anticonvulsants: midazolam or diazepam 0.5 mg/kg IV; intravenous lipid emulsion; oxygen administration
	Excessive plasma concentration (dose dependent), also related to potency of local anesthetic drug	Unconsciousness, coma	Stop administration of local anesthetic, continuous monitoring of ECG, monitor ventilation, airway maintenance, oxygen supplementation, epinephrine, intravenous fluids, intravenous lipid emulsion
	Excessive plasma concentration (dose dependent), also related to potency of local anesthetic drug	Respiratory arrest	Stop administration of local anesthetic, intubation and oxygen supplementation, ventilation, intravenous lipid emulsion
Neurotoxicity	Rare complication. Direct exposure of nerves to local anesthetics can result in toxicity of neural fibers, leading to concentration- dependent nerve damage and decreased neural blood flow. More likely to see neurotoxicity with spinals and epidurals. Return to normal function may occur over time	Pain, motor or sensory deficits, urinary or fecal incontinence	Stop administration of local anesthetic, supportive care, systemic analgesics for pain

References

Lin, Y. & Liu, S.S. (2013) Local anesthetics. In: Barasch, P.G., Cullen, B.F., Sotelting, R.K., et al. (eds) *Clinical Anesthesia*, 7th edn. Philadelphia: Lippincott Williams & Wilkins, pp.561–577.

Salinas, F.V., Liu, S.L. & Scholz, A.M. (2004) Analgesics: ion channel ligands/sodium channel blockers/local anesthetics. In: Evers, A.S. & Maze, M. (eds) *Anesthetic Pharmacology: Physiologic Principles and Clinical Practice*. Philadelphia: Churchill Livingstone, pp.507–533.

Stoelting, R.K. & Hillier, S.C. (2006) Local anesthetics. In: Stoelting, R.K. & Hillier, S.C. (eds) *Pharmacology & Physiology in Anesthetic Practice*, 4th edn. Philadelphia: Lippincott Williams & Wilkins, pp.179–207.

Weinberg, G., Ripper, R., Feinstein, D.L., et al. (2003) Lipid emulsion infusion rescues dogs from bupivacaine-induced cardiac toxicity. *Reg Anesth Pain Med* **28**: 198–202.

Further reading

Martin-Flores, M. (2013) Clinical pharmacology and toxicology of local anesthetic and adjuncts. In: Campoy, L. & Read, M.R. (eds) *Small Animal Regional Anesthesia and Analgesia*. Ames, IA: Wiley-Blackwell, pp.25–38.

Skarda, R.T. & Tranquilli, W.J. (2007) Local anesthetics. In: Tranquilli, W.J., Thurmon, J.C. & Grimm, K.A. (eds) *Lumb & Jones' Veterinary Anesthesia and Analgesia*, 4th edn. Ames, IA: Wiley-Blackwell, pp.395–418.

Index